Presented to:

_____

From:

_____

Date:

_____

DR. CHERRY'S
Little Instruction Book

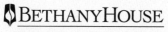
BETHANYHOUSE
MINNEAPOLIS, MN 55438

Dr. Cherry's Little Instruction Book
Copyright © 1999, 2003
Reginald B. Cherry. M.D.

Scripture credits are on page 155.

Cover design by Cheryl Neisen

The directions given in this book are in no way to be
considered a substitute for consultation with your own
physician.

Published by Bethany House Publishers
A Ministry of Bethany Fellowship International
11400 Hampshire Avenue South
Bloomington, Minnesota 55438
www.bethanyhouse.com

Printed in the United States of America by
Bethany Press International, Bloomington, Minnesota 55438

ISBN 0-7642-2768-8

Introduction

It is our vision to bring health and healing to the entire body of Christ. Second Corinthians 4:7 says that the treasure we have is contained in an earthen vessel. That treasure within us is the light and the anointing of God. When this earthen vessel is weakened by sickness and disease, that precious anointing cannot go forth and touch the hurting world around us with the good news of Jesus.

In these last days the evil one, who is the source of all disease, is not so much interested in attacking our physical bodies as that treasure contained in our earthen vessel. If the enemy can cripple and disable our physical bodies, he can quench the anointing that is within and prevent us from going into "all the world" and being a "light set on a hill." (See Mark 16:15 and Matthew 5:14.)

Dr. Cherry's Little Instruction Book on health and healing is meant to serve as a starting point for you to find your personal pathway to healing, so that you can defeat the enemy.

God still heals His people supernaturally just as He healed blind Bartimaeus in Mark 10. However, God's healing anointing also flows through natural substances just as He healed the blind man in John 9:6–7 through the use of natural substances (mud and saliva). Just as he was healed as he "went his way," so too there is a unique healing pathway for each of you, your family, and your brothers and sisters in the body of Christ.

HEALING IS OFTEN A PROCESS: AS WE DO WHAT WE CAN DO IN THE NATURAL, GOD WILL DO WHAT WE CANNOT DO IN THE SUPERNATURAL.

Dr. Cherry's Little Instruction Book

STEPS TOWARD WALKING IN YOUR PATHWAY TO HEALING:

- *Find out all you can do in the natural. Set yourself in agreement with God's Word.*

- *Exercise your faith knowing that the blood of the Lamb healed you two thousand years ago as Jesus bore your infirmities in His own body.*

PRINCIPLES OF PRAYING FOR HEALING

Thoughts: We must get our thinking right to fight off disease. You must start by saturating your mind with love. Read 1 Corinthians 13:4–8 daily. Love casts out fear and enables your faith to work. Learn to think on the right things; read Philippians 4:8.

Attitude: You must have a fighting attitude toward disease in your body. Matthew 11:12 says, ". . . the violent take it by force."

Talking Right: Convert your thoughts into words. Read Mark 11:23, Exodus 15:26, Isaiah 53:3–5, Matthew 8:17, and 1 Peter 2:24.

Know Whom You Are Fighting Against: Ephesians 6:12 says we don't wrestle against flesh and blood, but against principalities and powers of darkness.

Dr. Cherry's Little Instruction Book

SEVEN WAYS TO A HEALTHY LIFE

1. *Guard your heart and vascular system.*
2. *Protect yourself against cancer.*
3. *Balance your immune system.*
4. *Take recommended supplements.*
5. *Eat properly.*
6. *Exercise regularly.*
7. *Deal with stress.*

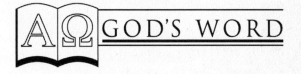

GOD'S WORD

I will praise thee; for I am fearfully and wonderfully made: marvellous are thy works; and that my soul knoweth right well.

—Psalm 139:14

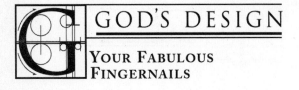

GOD'S DESIGN

YOUR FABULOUS FINGERNAILS

Doctors are taught in medical school to examine the fingernails. Why? Because with the exception of the eye, there is no part of the human body from which we can discover so many signs of disease. The fingernails, one of God's created wonders, serve as "windows" to examine so many other parts of the body.

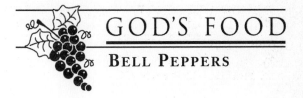

GOD'S FOOD

BELL PEPPERS

Bell pepper ranks near the top of the list when rated by the number of nutrients per calorie. Its most impressive characteristic is its extremely high vitamin C content.

The vitamin C content of peppers doubles when they're ripe, so use red bell peppers when available. To preserve vitamin C, peppers should be kept chilled, heated rapidly, and cooked the shortest time possible (or not at all!).

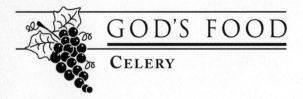

GOD'S FOOD

CELERY

Celery is high in the chemical apigenin, which can dilate blood vessels. Studies have indicated that it can also help with blood pressure. Celery also contains a chemical very similar to the prescription drugs known as calcium blockers and, therefore, is useful for some people who have irregular heartbeats.

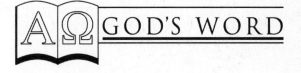

GOD'S WORD

I will pray with the spirit, and I will pray with the understanding also.

—1 Corinthians 14:15

Whosoever shall say unto this mountain, Be thou removed, and be thou cast into the sea . . . he shall have whatsoever he saith.

—Mark 11:23

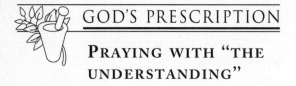

GOD'S PRESCRIPTION

PRAYING WITH "THE UNDERSTANDING"

Praying with "the understanding" means we understand what the enemy's attack is against our body and speak to our specific mountain according to what Jesus declared. We are now praying what James calls an effective prayer.

The effectual fervent prayer of a righteous man availeth much.

—James 5:16

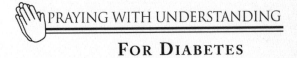 PRAYING WITH UNDERSTANDING

FOR DIABETES

Father, in the name of Jesus, I speak to the receptor cells in this body. I command them to become more sensitive and less resistant to the effects of insulin, allowing glucose to enter my body cells, supply energy, and perform the other functions of glucose.

Father, in the name of Jesus, I speak to the beta cells of my pancreas and command them to secrete adequate and normal amounts of insulin. I believe, Father, that my blood sugar levels will drop and my arteries, nerves, and eyes will be protected from destruction caused by high blood-sugar levels.

Father, I ask you to help me do my part by

maintaining my normal weight and eating the proper foods as I avoid simple carbo-hydrates and consume more fiber.

Father, reveal to me all of the things in the natural that I can do such as taking supple-ments and eating the right foods to take care of this temple. As I do those things I can do in the natural, I will believe and look to you to perform the supernatural in protecting all of the parts of my body from the effects of diabetes as my insulin levels become normal and my blood-sugar levels drop.

Thank you, Lord God, that I was healed of this disease by the blood of Jesus two thou-sand years ago, and therefore I am praying for the full manifestation of total healing in my body because by His stripes I was healed (1 Peter 2:24).

In Jesus' name, I pray. Amen.

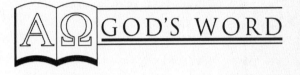

GOD'S WORD

And ye shall serve the LORD your God, and he shall bless thy bread, and thy water; and I will take sickness away from the midst of thee.

—Exodus 23:25

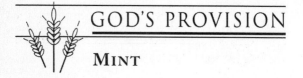

GOD'S PROVISION

MINT

Mint has several antioxidants that can help in protecting from both heart disease and cancer. Mint also contains selenium, which helps strengthen immune system function, and several antiviral compounds, many of which can target the herpes virus, which can cause fever blisters and other infections.

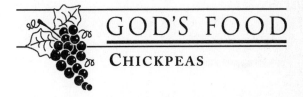

GOD'S FOOD
CHICKPEAS

Chickpeas are popular in countries like India. They have significant amounts of fiber, protein, iron, and potassium, as well as niacin. Studies show that chickpeas can have a significant lowering effect on cholesterol. Chickpeas also contain natural phytoestrogens, which can help prevent breast cancer in women and protect men from prostate cancer.

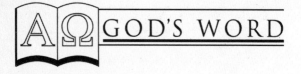

GOD'S WORD

And God said, Behold, I have given you every herb bearing seed, which is upon the face of all the earth, and every tree, in the which is the fruit of a tree yielding seed; to you it shall be for meat. . . . Every moving thing that liveth shall be meat for you; even as the green herb have I given you all things.

—Genesis 1:29; 9:3

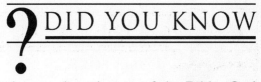

? DID YOU KNOW

In the very last chapter of the Bible, God reveals ". . . and the leaves of the tree were for the healing of the nations" (Revelation 22:2). In fact, of all the laws that God gave His people, one in every three relates to health. Science continues to confirm the truth of God's nutritional laws.

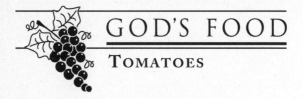

GOD'S FOOD

TOMATOES

Tomatoes contain one of the most potent cancer-fighting compounds known. The red tint in tomatoes is attributed to a potent compound known as lycopene. Even common ketchup contains this compound, as do all of the soups, casseroles, sauces, and relishes made with tomatoes. Lycopene is actually a carotenoid, which is the family that also contains beta-carotene.

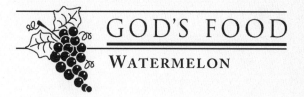

GOD'S FOOD
WATERMELON

Watermelon, like tomatoes, is high in lycopene. It has somewhat lesser amounts of lycopene than tomatoes, but also provides moderate amounts of vitamin C, beta-carotene, and potassium as well as small amounts of dietary fiber.

The ideal watermelon should be somewhat heavy for its size and should be symmetrical, that is it should be the same on each end and each side. The underside of a ripe watermelon should be pale or creamy yellow.

? DID YOU KNOW

Jesus told us in John 14 that He would ". . . pray the Father, and he shall give you another Comforter" and in John 16, ". . . He will guide you into all truth." Even with the increasingly complex diagnostic medical equipment available to doctors, no medical device or physician can diagnose a medical problem as well as the Holy Spirit, as He guides us to all truth!

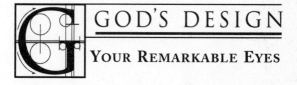

GOD'S DESIGN

YOUR REMARKABLE EYES

Nowhere in the human body is the wonderful design of our Creator better illustrated than in the eye. The Bible talks about the eye being "the light of the body" (Matthew 6:22) in the spiritual sense, but it also serves as a window to the physical body. Over two hundred different diseases throughout the body can be diagnosed by examining the eye! There is no camera or camcorder in the world that can even come close to the function of the human eye.

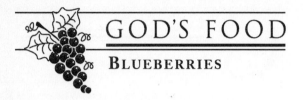

GOD'S FOOD

BLUEBERRIES

Blueberries are the subject of extensive research by scientists. It seems that the dye contained in the skin of blueberries has unusual beneficial qualities. To scientists these dyes are known as anthocyanins, which is from a Greek word for "dark blue." Anthocyanins have recently been discovered to protect not only the heart and other body tissues, but also the brain.

A recent research study revealed that among forty fruits and vegetables tested, blueberries had the highest antioxidant capacity because of the large amount of anthocyanins.

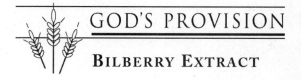

GOD'S PROVISION

BILBERRY EXTRACT

Bilberry extract comes from a small European blueberry and is available over the counter without a prescription. The pigment in their skin and also in the pulp part of the berry is more potent than blueberries. Bilberry extract has almost the identical amount of protective antioxidants as fresh blueberries.

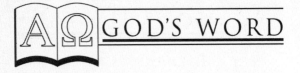

GOD'S WORD

If thou wilt diligently hearken to the voice of the LORD thy God, and wilt do that which is right in his sight ...I will put [allow] none of these diseases upon thee ... for I am the LORD that healeth thee.

—Exodus 15:26

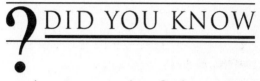

? DID YOU KNOW

Research points out that God may have already warned us about the cause of some diseases thirty-five centuries ago: "It shall be a perpetual statute for your generations throughout all your dwellings, that ye eat neither fat nor blood" (Leviticus 3:17).

In these simple Scriptures, God warns the Israelites against consuming certain types of fats, particularly saturated fats from animals. Even though the Israelites ate animal meat, it was wild meat and contained *omega-3 fatty acids* similar to that found in salmon and mackerel today.

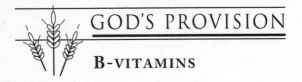

GOD'S PROVISION

B-VITAMINS

B-vitamins: Simple supplementation with a vitamin such as B-100 complex would provide all of the B-vitamins, including folic acid (a synthetic form of folate), B_6, and B_{12}. All of these B-vitamins lower the levels of homocysteine in the blood and offer protection from heart disease, stroke, and possibly Alzheimer's disease.

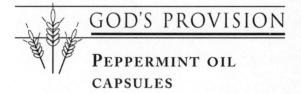

GOD'S PROVISION

PEPPERMINT OIL CAPSULES

Peppermint oil capsules have been used for several years in Europe for the treatment of irritable bowel syndrome and have been found to be very safe and effective. The oil appears to stop excessive contraction of smooth muscles and helps maintain the muscle tone in the colon. One to two capsules daily between meals would be the recommended treatment if you are suffering from irritability or spasms in the colon.

PRAYING WITH UNDERSTANDING

FOR IMMUNE SYSTEM DISEASES

Father, I come before you in the mighty name of Jesus. I thank you, Father, that Your Son, Jesus, bore in His own body two thousand years ago on Calvary every immune system disease. Therefore, I thank you that by His stripes I was healed. I come before you seeking total and complete healing for my immune system.

I speak, Father, in the name of Jesus to the components of my immune system that are mistakenly attacking my own body. I command my immune system to recognize the normal components in my body, and I speak balance to the immune cells. I speak protection over my heart, my lungs, my joints, my kidneys, and every cell, organ, and blood vessel in my body.

I ask you, Father, to show me the specific pathway that will lead to total healing in my body. Reveal through the leading of the Holy Spirit those natural substances that I can take that will balance my immune system.

Father, I look to you to do the supernatural to produce the full manifestation of healing in my temple. I thank you, Father, that according to 1 Peter 2:24 I was healed, and I thank you that the full, complete, and total manifestation of that healing is mine. Through my eye of faith I see myself healed. I thank you, Father, for this healing manifestation.

In the precious name of Jesus. Amen.

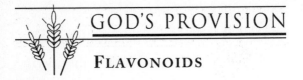

GOD'S PROVISION

FLAVONOIDS

Flavonoids are nutrients that occur naturally in various plants such as tea, fruits, and vegetables. God created flavonoids to protect us from and fight diseases ranging from cancer to heart disease, circulatory problems, and attention deficit disorder. There are many different kinds of flavonoids.

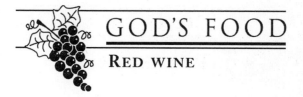

GOD'S FOOD
RED WINE

Red wine is a rich source of the flavonoid known as proanthocyanidin, which helps prevent platelets in the blood from sticking to artery walls, causing dangerous blood clots. This flavonoid has been shown to offer protection from heart disease, cancer, and even stroke.

Research has shown that the French, who consume wine as a staple, have lower rates of heart disease even though their typical diet is high in fat. Fortunately, there are now alcohol-free red wines available, which provide us with all the benefits of wine without the detrimental effects of alcohol.

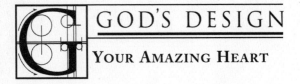

GOD'S DESIGN

YOUR AMAZING HEART

God designed the heart to function in a majestic, orderly pattern, and He has revealed His design to us. By careful examination of the heart, we can detect minute deviations from God's design that give us important clues to problems that may be developing with the heart.

? DID YOU KNOW

Remarkably, the heart can keep on beating even if all the other nerves are severed. With each beat, the average adult heart pumps out about 4 ounces of blood, which adds up to 3,000 gallons per day or over 1,095,000 gallons a year. That's enough to fill more than 46 railroad tank cars with 23,000 gallons each.

The heart works hard enough in one hour to lift a 150-pound man to the top of a three-story building. There's enough energy created by the heart to lift a 65-ton tank car one foot off the ground, and enough power generated by a single heart in 70 years to lift the largest battleship afloat completely out of the water!

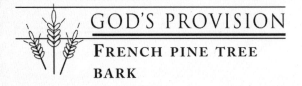

GOD'S PROVISION
FRENCH PINE TREE BARK

French pine tree bark, which has been used for centuries, also contains powerful flavonoids, proanthocyanidins. These chemical compounds protect the body's cells and help protect against degenerative diseases, heart disease, and stroke. Grape seeds also contain the same compound. These protective compounds have been patented and made available in a supplement form known as Pycnogenol.

Also, pine bark can increase fertility in both normal and infertile men. The extract from the pine tree bark has also been used to treat attention deficit disorder (ADD) and attention deficit/hyperactivity disorder (ADHD).

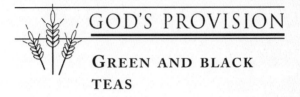

GOD'S PROVISION

GREEN AND BLACK TEAS

Green and black teas are excellent sources of flavonoids known as catechins. Green tea, which is a nonfermented tea, is richer in these protective substances. Studies in Japan indicate they offer protection from numerous diseases including cancer, heart disease, and stroke, as well as several cancers of the GI tract, including stomach and esophageal cancer.

? DID YOU KNOW

Did you know God has provided many ways for us to prevent disease in these last days? It's true. An example may be found with one of the most common diseases facing the modern world—hardening of the arteries and heart disease.

A survey taken among members of the American College of Cardiology found that the most common preventive used by cardiologists themselves is the antioxidant vitamin E. Other supplements that cardiologists take are vitamin C and beta carotene. Many cardiologists also take a daily aspirin as a preventive.

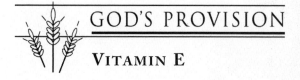

GOD'S PROVISION

Vitamin E

Vitamin E prevents the oxidation of bad (LDL) cholesterol. LDL cholesterol must first be oxidized before it can deposit in the arteries and lead to blockage. Although vitamin E can be obtained from many foods, it is much easier to take a supplement. When you buy vitamin E, simply look on the label for the word "natural." The natural form is more potent than the synthetic form.

Amazingly, the American Heart Association has cited vitamin E as one of the "top ten heart and stroke research advances." God's creation of this remarkable vitamin has provided us with a wonderful preventive for many diseases!

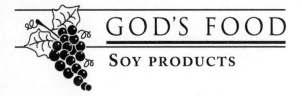

GOD'S FOOD

SOY PRODUCTS

Soy products contain a potent type of flavonoid known as isoflavones. Because of the high isoflavone activity, soy products produce a mild estrogenic effect in the human body and can protect women from breast cancer, heart disease, and osteoporosis; they can also ease the symptoms of menopause.

Soy can be found in many forms: drink mixes, tofu, soy powders, soy milk, and protein bars.

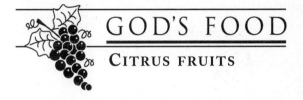

GOD'S FOOD

CITRUS FRUITS

Citrus fruits also contain many different types of flavonoids. Dr. Fotsis at the University of Ioannina in Greece found that certain citric flavonoids actually cut off the blood supply to tumors. Research in Japan has identified two flavonoids (*diosmin* and *hesperidin*) that are especially effective against cancer in the oral cavity.

Oranges, grapefruit, tangerines, lemons, and limes are common citrus fruits, but for variety try these lesser known citrus fruits—kumquats, pomelos, and tangelos.

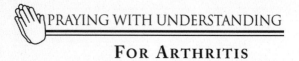

PRAYING WITH UNDERSTANDING

FOR ARTHRITIS

Father, I come before you in the name of your precious Son, Jesus, thanking you that Jesus bore the symptoms of the infirmity of arthritis in His own body 2,000 years ago. I thank you that because He bore this disease in His own body, I was healed!

Therefore, Father, I am coming before you seeking the manifestation of that healing in my physical body. In the name of Jesus, I speak to the cartilage in my joints [name the joint where you are suffering pain], and I command that cartilage to increase in thickness and become more pliable and more elastic.

I further pray that the inflammatory cells

that lead to swelling and pain be removed from that joint. In Jesus' name, I confess that I will be able to move that joint and serve you day to day without pain, symptoms, or inflammation in my body.

Father, as I do all I can do in the natural, I look to you to do the supernatural in me that I cannot do. I ask you to send forth the healing, anointing power of the Holy Spirit into my body and into my joints, and I speak comfort and healing to these joints.

Thank you, Father, that my manifestation of healing is on the way. I praise you, Father, that you are revealing the specific pathway that will lead to my healing. I thank you for all of these things in the precious name of Jesus, and I close this prayer praising and thanking you because through my eyes of faith, I see myself healed.

In Jesus' name, amen.

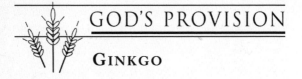

GOD'S PROVISION

GINKGO

Ginkgo has been in the news lately. It is a potent *flavonoid* credited with increasing circulation in the brain, reducing short-term memory loss, and helping with circulatory problems in the extremities. A recent study in the *Journal of the American Medical Association* found that ginkgo improves blood flow into the brain and can improve the symptoms of Alzheimer's disease.

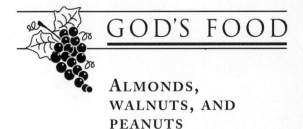

GOD'S FOOD

ALMONDS, WALNUTS, AND PEANUTS

Almonds, walnuts, and peanuts provide numerous healing and protective benefits. A recent study released in the *British Medical Journal* shows that regular consumption of nuts leads to a 35 percent drop in the risk of having a heart attack.

Nuts contain significant amounts of magnesium, vitamin E, potassium, and alpha-linoleic acid, all of which benefit the coronary arteries. Consistently, people who consume large amounts of nuts, such as almonds, have significant reductions in blood cholesterol. Since they are derived from plants, they contain no cholesterol at all.

? DID YOU KNOW

Nuts are very high in fat (the good kind of fat) and are thus high in calories. So plan your consumption of nuts carefully. I personally recommend plain, unsalted almonds—ten daily. Recent studies show they will drop cholesterol as well as prescription medicine. Moderation is the key. I encourage you to begin consuming small amounts of nuts daily, especially almonds.

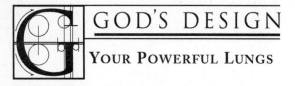

GOD'S DESIGN
YOUR POWERFUL LUNGS

God designed our lungs both to rid our bodies of harmful waste products (such as carbon dioxide) and to supply our red blood cells with fresh oxygen, enabling normal cell function and proper metabolism.

GOD'S PRESCRIPTION

HOW TO QUIT SMOKING

- Pick a date to quit (about two weeks away); either quit cold turkey or begin tapering.
- Throw away ALL of your cigarettes.
- When you feel the urge to smoke, remember the 4 Ds—**Delay, Deep breathing, Drink** (1–2 glasses of water), and **Do** something else.
- Exercise! Remember the irritability, tiredness, trouble sleeping, coughing, or depression will all disappear.
- Avoid sugar, drink plenty of water, and try low-calorie snacks (popcorn, raw veggies).

Ask your doctor about a skin patch, gum,

or other aid designed to help you win the
victory over cigarettes.

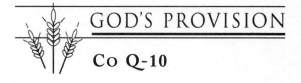

GOD'S PROVISION

Co Q-10

Co Q-10 is an antioxidant and thus, can have cancer and heart disease protective effects.

Dr. Langsjoen, a physician in Texas, has done a great deal of research on Co Q-10 and has found that Co Q-10 can significantly decrease the symptoms of congestive heart failure such as shortness of breath, fluid buildup in the lower extremities, and inability to lie flat.

More recently, researchers have used Co Q-10 in the treatment of cancer. It appears to benefit cancer patients by enhancing immune system function.

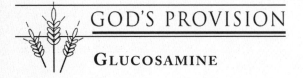

GOD'S PROVISION

GLUCOSAMINE

Glucosamine has been proven to be as effective as prescription medicine for osteo-arthritis (the most common form of arthritis). This natural substance, which is produced in the body, stimulates the repair of cartilage while reducing inflammation in the joint. It often takes two to three months before the effects occur, but this natural pathway, combined with the power of prayer, has actually prevented joint replacement surgeries.

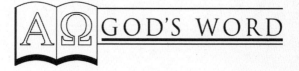

GOD'S WORD

One of the most astounding and eye-opening Scriptures in the Bible is found in Proverbs 18:9. *The Amplified Bible* reads, "He who does not use his endeavors to heal himself is brother to him who commits suicide."

? DID YOU KNOW

We often allow depression into our lives, not from an attack of the enemy, but simply because we do not follow God's Word and apply Scriptures such as 1 Peter 5:7, where we are instructed to cast our care on Him, "Casting all your care upon him; for he careth for you."

God has also provided us with various natural substances (such as Saint-John's-wort, valerian, and other substances) to help restore these chemical levels to normal as we begin applying the Word of God and prayer in the supernatural realm.

PRAYING WITH UNDERSTANDING

FOR DEPRESSION

Thank you, Father, that I can come into your presence in the name of your precious Son, Jesus. I thank You, Father, that Jesus bore in His body all of my infirmities and all of my iniquities, and this includes the depression that I am experiencing.

Since I have been healed of this according to 1 Peter 2:24, I now seek you for the unique pathway that will lead to the total and complete manifestation of my healing. Through the Holy Spirit, Father, reveal to me all the things I can do in the natural to overcome this attack.

As I do all I can do, Lord, I look to you to do the supernatural that I cannot do. I speak to the neurotransmitter chemicals in my brain and I command them to be normal in the name of Jesus. I thank you, Father, that I have the mind of Christ and that my thoughts will be clear and all symptoms of depression will go.

I call myself healed and through my eye of faith, I see myself healed, and I believe that the full manifestation of my healing is on the way. I believe, Father, that you will satisfy me with long life and fulfill the number of my days. I thank you that I have authority over the power of darkness, and in Jesus' name I execute that authority and command the grip of darkness to be released from my mind in Jesus' name.

Thank you, Father, that it is done and as I am set free of this depression, I will find, follow, and complete your divine will for my life.

In Jesus' name I pray, amen.

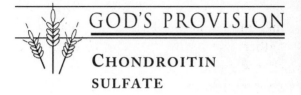

GOD'S PROVISION

CHONDROITIN SULFATE

Chondroitin sulfate is naturally produced in the body and helps make the cartilage that lines the joints more elastic by causing increased water retention. It can also block enzymes that tend to destroy cartilage. Both glucosamine and chondroitin sulfate are natural, very safe, and are available at health food stores.

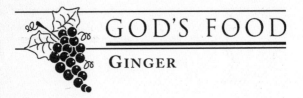

GOD'S FOOD
GINGER

Ginger has been consumed for thousands of years to help treat dizziness. In one study of sailors consuming one gram of powdered ginger two to three times daily, there were markedly reduced symptoms associated with seasickness, such as vomiting and dizziness.

Ginger is also available in capsules and can be taken thirty minutes before dizziness might be anticipated and then every one to two hours.

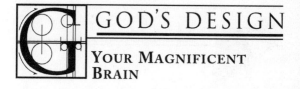

GOD'S DESIGN

YOUR MAGNIFICENT BRAIN

Our brain is so wonderfully made, and God worked out a marvelous plan to maintain healthy brain function through various foods that we eat. By eating the right foods, brain and memory function can be restored and maintained to a ripe old age.

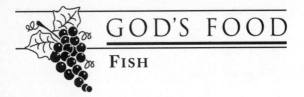

GOD'S FOOD

FISH

Fish has long been considered "brain food." Scientists are continually confirming this. Sardines are not usually associated with an improvement in brain function, but they provide an omega-3 fatty acid (found also in deepwater fish such as salmon) that can decrease the inflammatory processes that occur in the brain with aging. Sardines also supply substances that can be converted into choline to make acetylcholine, which is essential for proper brain function.

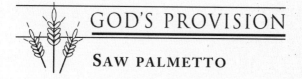

GOD'S PROVISION

SAW PALMETTO

Saw palmetto has become known as a natural, plant-derived treatment for symptoms of an enlarged prostate. We have now discovered that extracts from another plant (pygeum) can have a similar beneficial effect, and in fact, the two extracts can be taken together for added benefits.

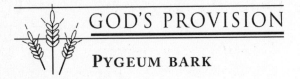

GOD'S PROVISION

PYGEUM BARK

Pygeum bark contains the chemical beta-sitosterol. Beta-sitosterol reduces inflammation, swelling, and edema (fluid accumulation) in the prostate gland. In addition to these benefits, many studies indicate significant improvements in various urinary tract symptoms. In fact, extracts from pygeum bark have been shown to be as effective as prescription medications.

Dr. Cherry's Little Instruction Book

DR. CHERRY'S TOP 10 WAYS TO PREVENT BREAST CANCER

1. *Consume soy and isoflavones.*
2. *Add cold-water fish to your diet.*
3. *Eat kiwifruit.*
4. *Eat 10 almonds and 5 prunes a day.*
5. *Eat oranges.*
6. *Take psyllium.*
7. *Cook with olive oil.*
8. *Eat cabbage and broccoli.*
9. *Enjoy yogurt.*
10. *Take vitamin A (beta carotene).*

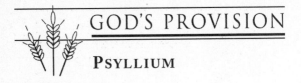

GOD'S PROVISION

PSYLLIUM

Psyllium is a common laxative that can also lower your cholesterol level. Psyllium products are actually forms of soluble fiber similar to those found in apples, beans, etc.

Psyllium could reduce your risk of heart attack by up to 25 percent. It acts like a sponge to soak up cholesterol (bile acids) in the intestine and causes the liver to remove cholesterol from the blood. It also may decrease the risk of colon cancer by expelling toxic bile acids, and it protects against diverticulosis by softening stools.

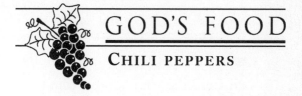

GOD'S FOOD
CHILI PEPPERS

Chili peppers are helpful in the treatment of depression. They increase the level of endorphins in the brain. Endorphins elevate mood. Did you know that some people get hooked on chili peppers, eating stronger and stronger chili peppers because of this endorphin release? Don't overdo a good thing!

? DID YOU KNOW

Research from the University of Illinois at Chicago showed that a component of grapes known as *resveratrol* could actually inhibit the growth of tumors. Resveratrol inhibits tumor growth at three different stages (initiation, promotion, and progression).

Throughout the Bible, we see so many references to grapes and grape-related products (e.g., wine: Matthew 26:29; Mark 14:25; Luke 22:18), so it makes us wonder if God had something special in mind when He created this fruit.

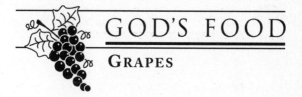

GOD'S FOOD
GRAPES

Grapes contain resveratrol, which attacks two of our biggest killers: cancer and heart disease. Grapes also contain chemicals that can prevent blood clots and can inhibit breast, liver, and colon cancer. They help prevent heart attacks by preventing cholesterol from depositing in the arteries. Resveratrol also stimulates and helps nerve cells to regenerate.

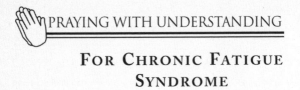

PRAYING WITH UNDERSTANDING

FOR CHRONIC FATIGUE SYNDROME

Father, I come to you in the name of Jesus, thanking you that Jesus bore in His own body on the cross two thousand years ago the infirmity of chronic fatigue syndrome that has attacked my body. I therefore pray, Father, asking you to guide me to the pathway that will lead to the total manifestation of my healing.

In the name of Jesus, I speak to my immune system, and I command it to become balanced according to the Word of God and according to the way you created it to function. I speak to any abnormal chemical levels in my body and command them to also become normal. I command the ATP levels that produce energy in my body to become normal in Jesus' name.

I thank you, Father, that as I do my part and balance my immune system with the natural substances you created, that you will supernaturally touch and heal me of this attack of darkness. I thank you, Lord, for revelation knowledge of new chemicals discovered in your creation that will help set me free.

Thank you, Father, that there is a unique pathway for me to walk on, and as I am obedient and go my way I will be set free and will be satisfied with long life on this earth according to your promise. In Jesus' name, I thank you that my healing is coming, and through my eye of faith, I see myself healed.

In Jesus' name, amen.

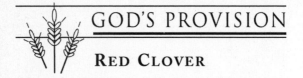

GOD'S PROVISION

RED CLOVER

Red clover is the source of a natural plant-derived estrogen. A study published in *The Journal of Clinical Endocrinology and Metabolism* reveals how derivations from red clover can maintain normal estrogen levels in women, reduce or prevent hot flashes, maintain elasticity in blood vessels, and in general, protect women from the effects of menopause.

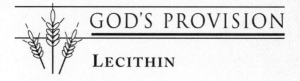

GOD'S PROVISION

LECITHIN

Lecithin is an over-the-counter supplement that is high in choline, one of the B-vitamins. It can improve memory function. Granules of lecithin can be used on cereals and other foods to help the body produce more acetylcholine. Low levels of acetylcholine are associated with age-related memory impairment.

Phosphatidylserine is a concentrated component of lecithin and can improve brain function even in the early stages of Alzheimer's disease. In healthy persons, it can improve concentration and the ability to recall names and other details.

? DID YOU KNOW

Scientists have once again turned to God's plant kingdom and found some incredible substances that will now be added to a food (in this case, margarine) and will help significantly lower cholesterol levels. One of the substances comes from soybean oil extract and the other comes from pine trees!

The stanol-based healthy margarine (Benecol) has been shown to lower total cholesterol by 10% and the LDL blood levels (bad cholesterol) by 14%. The plant sterol-based margarine (Take Control) has been shown to lower the bad cholesterol by 7 to 10%. These percentage numbers may not seem very high, but remember that a 10% drop in total cholesterol equals a 20% decrease in the risk of coronary artery disease.

? DID YOU KNOW

Can you believe that "designer eggs" are starting to appear on supermarket shelves? Scientists have discovered that changing the diet of hens can markedly increase the eggs' content of omega-3 fatty acids (especially DHA), which can have great benefit for the eyes, brain, and heart. The omega-3 fatty acids can lower the rate of heart disease, help with manic-depressive problems, prevent cardiac irregularities, and help with inflammatory colon problems. In addition, hens on the special diet are producing eggs with six times the amount of vitamin E content of regular eggs.

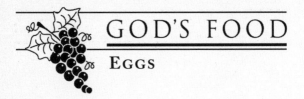

GOD'S FOOD
EGGS

Eggs are a good source of choline and B-vitamins and, of course, are high in protein also. Protein intake early in the day helps us feel more alert by affecting brain chemical levels. And although eggs are a concentrated source of cholesterol, it is not the cholesterol intake in our diet that contributes to heart problems, but it is primarily the saturated fat intake that is the problem.

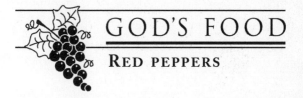

GOD'S FOOD

RED PEPPERS

Red peppers can protect brain function because they contain carotinoids and vitamin C, which help provide antioxidants. Higher levels of vitamin C in the bloodstream have been positively associated with improved memory.

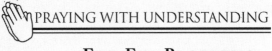

PRAYING WITH UNDERSTANDING

FOR EYE PROBLEMS

Father, as I come before you in the name of your precious Son, Jesus, I thank you for the divine health that He purchased for me on Calvary. I thank you, Father, that Jesus gave us the authority of His name and the anointing of the Holy Spirit to overcome the works of the enemy that attack my body.

Father, I thank you for divine eyesight and clear vision. I thank you, Father, for protecting the lens of my eye from cataracts. I command nutrients and antioxidants and protective chemicals in my blood to flow in and touch the lens of my eye and protect it from degenerative changes. As I place these nutrients into my body, I thank you, Father, that they will go forth and accomplish the purpose for which you created them.

I further thank you, Father, that the pressure within my eye will be normal and glaucoma will not be allowed to exist within my eye and cause damage.

I thank you, Father, that I will continue to have sharp, clear vision and will not suffer the effects of macular degeneration. I speak to the pigments that you created in the area of my retina, and I command them to increase. Thank you, Father, that my vision will be sharp and focused. I will eat those substances and take in those nutrients that will protect the macular area of my retina and I thank you, Father, that dimmed vision and blindness will not exist in this temple.

In Jesus' name, I praise you for all of these things. Amen.

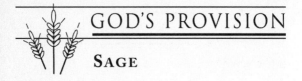

GOD'S PROVISION

SAGE

Sage is a popular herb used in cooking, but it also inhibits a certain enzyme that breaks down the acetylcholine levels in the brain. By raising acetylcholine levels, memory can be improved. Sage should be used as much as possible in cooking because of this protective action.

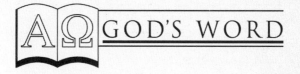

GOD'S WORD

Is anyone among you sick? Let him call for the elders of the church, and let them pray over him, anointing him with oil in the name of the Lord. And the prayer of faith will save the sick, and the Lord will raise him up. And if he has committed sins, he will be forgiven.

—James 5:14–15 NKJV

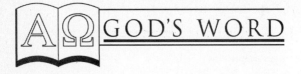 GOD'S WORD

The Bible says that we have the power to add to or take away the number of our days (Proverbs 9:11). God also declares in Psalm 91:16 that He will satisfy us with long life. In Exodus 23:26, God promises that He will ". . . fulfill the number of our days."

Cling to these Scriptures and tie a satisfied long life with the call of God upon your life.

? DID YOU KNOW

A low-fat diet can fight arthritis. Several early findings have revealed some startling information. For example, researchers at Wayne State University Medical School evaluated patients with rheumatoid arthritis and placed them on a low-fat diet. In less than two months, all of the patients went into remission from the effects of rheumatoid arthritis. When fat was reintroduced to the diet, however, painful symptoms returned in only three days.

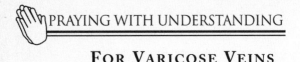

PRAYING WITH UNDERSTANDING

For Varicose Veins

Father, I come to you in the precious name of my Lord and Savior, Jesus. I thank you that He bore my infirmities on the cross two thousand years ago, and by His stripes I was healed. By the authority in that name, I speak to the veins in my legs and I command the valves in those veins to function normally.

I command the pressure in the veins and capillaries to decrease and the fluid leaking from those vessels to decrease and disappear. Furthermore, I take authority over the formation of any blood clot that might form in those veins and I say that my blood flow will be normal in Jesus' name.

I pray specifically for the Holy Spirit to guide me to the truth of my pathway to healing. If I am to use a natural treatment, I pray that your anointing will flow through the seed extract horsechestnut and those chemicals that you created within it will begin healing my veins. As I do the things in the natural that I have received knowledge of, I will trust you, Father, to do the supernatural that I cannot do. Thank you, Lord, for your hand of protection upon me, and I thank you that the full manifestation of healing is mine. Thank you, Father, for these things.

In Jesus' name, amen.

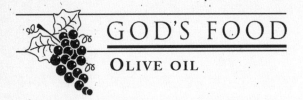

GOD'S FOOD

OLIVE OIL

Olive oil contains monounsaturated fats, which have significant heart benefits as well as cancer-protecting benefits. The oleic and steric acids help reduce the risk of breast cancer. Olive oil can be used alone on salads or mixed with vinegar for a simple dressing.

GOD'S FOOD

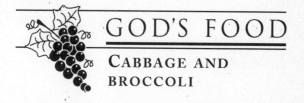

CABBAGE AND BROCCOLI

Cabbage and broccoli contain a chemical compound known as *indole-3-carbinol* that reduces the body's production of certain types of estrogen, which lead to breast cancer. Studies out of Cornell University Medical College reveal that these indoles also stop human breast cancer cells dead in their tracks. To get this protective substance, you should eat cabbage, broccoli, and brussels sprouts, as well as bok choy, chard, and turnips.

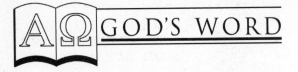

GOD'S WORD

In a spiritual sense, the Bible speaks frequently of God placing a "hedge of protection" around His people. In a natural sense, God has also created a "natural" hedge of protection inside the human body to protect us from a vast onslaught of diseases and illnesses. This natural hedge is known as the immune system.

Hast not thou made an hedge about him, and about his house . . . ?

—Job 1:10

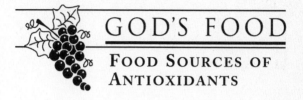

GOD'S FOOD

FOOD SOURCES OF ANTIOXIDANTS

Vitamin C: citrus fruits, strawberries, cantaloupe, broccoli, potatoes, tomatoes, and other fruits.

Vitamin E: vegetable oils, wheat germ, whole-grain bread and pasta.

Beta Carotene: broccoli, cantaloupe, carrots, spinach, squash, pumpkin, sweet potatoes, apricots, and other dark green, orange, and yellow vegetables.

Selenium: fish, meat, breads, and cereals.

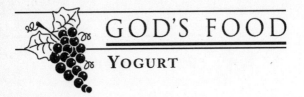

GOD'S FOOD
YOGURT

Yogurt contains large amounts of calcium, which can inhibit the division of breast cancer cells. Yogurt also stimulates gamma interferon, which helps fight cancer by enhancing immune system functions.

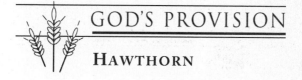

GOD'S PROVISION

HAWTHORN

Hawthorn has frequently been called a heart or cardiac tonic and has often been used with digoxin, which is another well-known treatment for congestive heart failure derived from the foxglove plant. Studies reveal numerous chemicals within the leaves, flowers, and berries of the hawthorn plant that strengthen the heart. The most potent of these chemicals occurs in the flowers.

Studies are now being conducted on hawthorn in mainstream medicine because of the beneficial effects on strengthening the heart.

DR. CHERRY'S TOP 12 WAYS TO BALANCE YOUR IMMUNE SYSTEM

1. *Vitamin E: helps preserve and strengthen the immune system function.*
2. *Multiple vitamin: a simple multiple vitamin is essential to maintain a complete balance in normal immune systems.*
3. *B Complex: vitamin B_6 has demonstrated a particularly strong positive effect on the immune system and is found in B-100 complex.*
4. *Vitamin C: has an important role in increasing the number of white blood cells, which form the backbone of our immune response.*
5. *Zinc: has long been known as an important substance in protecting the immune system. (Too much can be harmful, however. Only 15 mg. to 30 mg. a day is sufficient.)*

6. **Chromium:** has an indirect effect on the immune system by stimulating T-lymphocytes and interferon.

7. **Yogurt:** the live cultures in yogurt stimulate the immune system by causing the body to increase production of gamma interferon, which can fight off infections.

8. **Coenzyme Q-10:** studies show this can increase an important component of the immune system (gamma globulin).

9. **Garlic:** can stimulate and enhance the response of the immune system.

10. **Selenium:** can enhance immune system function, especially in fighting cancer. (Can be toxic in high doses; limit to 200 mcg. daily.)

11. **Echinacea:** this plant substance can also stimulate immune system function.

12. **Glutathione:** a potent antioxidant and immune system stimulant.

13 Best-Selling Herbs

1. **Chamomile:** *used as a tea, ointment, lotion, and as a mild sedative. It also seems to be effective in treating inflammation and spasms in the digestive track.*

But I will restore you to health and heal your wounds, declares the Lord.

—Jeremiah 30:17 NIV

13 BEST-SELLING HERBS

2. *Echinacea: has been shown to stimulate the immune system and is used for colds and flulike infections. Use only intermittently (8 weeks maximum, take 2 weeks off). The tincture is strongest; take 2–3 teaspoons daily.*

And the Lord will take away from thee all sickness, and will put none of the evil diseases of Egypt, which thou knowest, upon thee.

—Deuteronomy 7:15

13 BEST-SELLING HERBS

3. *Feverfew:* most promising use has been treating headaches, particularly migraines. It is also used for arthritis and stomach pain. Use the dry leaves (25 mg. twice daily), or the fluid extract (1/4–1/2 teaspoon three times daily).

I will not die but live, and will proclaim what the Lord has done.

—Psalm 118:17 NIV

13 BEST-SELLING HERBS

4. *Garlic: though not usually thought of as an herb, garlic is a bulbous herb that has demonstrated multiple benefits—fights bacteria, strengthens the immune system, raises the good cholesterol, and has potent cancer-fighting effects. Dried capsules equivalent to one clove of fresh garlic daily are suggested.*

Don't be afraid, for I am with you. Do not be dismayed, for I am your God. I will strengthen you. I will help you. I will uphold you with my victorious right hand.

—Isaiah 41:10 NLT

13 BEST-SELLING HERBS

5. *Ginger: used especially to prevent nausea and motion sickness and for digestion. May help fight colds. One gram of powdered root is typically taken two to three times daily.*

He himself bore our sins in his body on the tree, so that we might die to sins and live for righteousness; by his wounds you have been healed.

—1 Peter 2:24 NIV

13 BEST-SELLING HERBS

6. ***Ginkgo (biloba):*** *has been shown in many studies to improve circulation, especially to the brain, and therefore may improve short-term memory and treat headaches; it also may be beneficial in depression. Also functions as an antioxidant. Dose typically used is 40 mg. three times daily.*

For God hath not given us the spirit of fear; but of power, and of love, and of a sound mind.

—2 Timothy 1:7

13 Best-Selling Herbs

7. *Ginseng: has been recommended for increasing physical and mental capacities and to build up the body's resistance in times of stress. The data on ginseng is not as convincing as many other herbs, and there is much abuse in marketing this herb. More involved studies are currently in progress.*

Beat your plowshares into swords And your pruning hooks into spears; Let the weak say, "I am strong."

—Joel 3:10 NKJV

13 BEST-SELLING HERBS

8. ***Goldenseal:*** *tea used for respiratory problems and sinusitis; may fight certain bacterial and parasitic infections. Should not be taken for long periods of time (2 weeks maximum). Dosage would be tea 2–5 grams three times daily, or tincture (1:5) 1^{1}/$_{2}$–3 teaspoons three times daily.*

Dear friend, I am praying that all is well with you and that your body is as healthy as I know your soul is.

—3 John 2 NLT

13 BEST-SELLING HERBS

9. *Milk Thistle:* has been used in Europe to treat cirrhosis of the liver; helps liver cells rejuvenate in conditions such as jaundice or inflammation of liver cells due to content of the chemical silymarin. A standardized extract (70–210 mg.) three times daily has been used.

The power of the life-giving Spirit has freed you through Christ Jesus from the power of sin that leads to death.... The Spirit of God, who raised Jesus from the dead, lives in you. And just as he raised Christ from the dead, he will give life to your mortal body by this same Spirit living within you.

—Romans 8:2, 11 NLT

13 BEST-SELLING HERBS

10. ***Peppermint:*** *has been used for improving digestion, especially excessive gas. It is usually used as a tea, but exact beneficial dosage is not known.*

Don't worry about anything, but pray about everything. With thankful hearts offer up your prayers and requests to God. Then, because you belong to Christ Jesus, God will bless you with peace that no one can completely understand. And this peace will control the way you think and feel.

—Philippians 4:6–7 CEV

13 Best-Selling Herbs

11. ***Saw Palmetto:*** *this plant (seronoa repens) has been extensively used in Europe to treat enlarged prostate glands in men. Men experiencing difficulty in urination, slowness, or increased frequency should, of course, consult their doctor but might want to try 160 mg. twice daily.*

My son, give attention to my words; incline your ear to my sayings. Do not let them depart from your eyes; keep them in the midst of your heart; for they are life to those who find them, and health to all their flesh.

—Proverbs 4:20–22 NKJV

13 BEST-SELLING HERBS

12. ***Valerian:*** *may be useful as a minor tranquilizer and for sleep disorders. Can be taken as a tea (1–2 grams) 30 minutes before retiring, or fluid extract (¹/₂–1 teaspoon), or solid extract (250–500 mg.).*

Surely he hath borne our griefs, and carried our sorrows: yet we did esteem him stricken, smitten of God, and afflicted. But he was wounded for our transgressions, he was bruised for our iniquities: the chastisement of our peace was upon him; and with his stripes we are healed.

—Isaiah 53:4–5

13 BEST-SELLING HERBS

13. *Willowbark: widely used as a tea for headaches, fever, muscular pains, and arthritis. Contains salicylates, the active ingredient in aspirin.*

"Have faith in God," Jesus answered. "I tell you the truth, if anyone says to this mountain, 'Go, throw yourself into the sea,' and does not doubt in his heart but believes that what he says will happen, it will be done for him. Therefore I tell you, whatever you ask for in prayer, believe that you have received it, and it will be yours."

—Mark 11:22–24 NIV

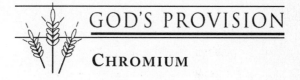

GOD'S PROVISION

CHROMIUM

Chromium can be used to maintain healthy glucose levels in the body. Studies demonstrating this have been reported in journals such as *Diabetic Medicine,* and more than 25 well-controlled clinical trials have taken place. Chromium apparently increases the ability of our body's insulin to be more effective, which in turn, may help many patients get off of diabetes medicine.

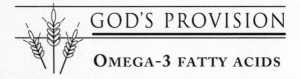

GOD'S PROVISION

OMEGA-3 FATTY ACIDS

Omega-3 fatty acids benefit the human body in many ways. They can protect women from breast cancer, ward off Alzheimer's disease, control diabetes, control high blood pressure, prevent a sudden heart attack, protect against ventricular fibrillation, reduce the risk of dying from heart disease, decrease the inflammation of rheumatoid arthritis, treat inflammation of the GI tract, fight depression and manic depressive illness, and help control attention deficit/hyper-activity disorder.

Omega-3s can be found in fish, flaxseed, canola, and walnuts, as well as dark green leafy vegetables. Fatty fish (salmon) are the best source.

DR. CHERRY'S TECHNIQUES FOR WEIGHT LOSS

Set a Realistic Goal—Don't set your goal too high; be realistic.

Avoid Deprivation—Extreme diets don't work. Compromise on portions instead.

Reduce Fat Intake—This is the number one way to long-term weight loss and maintenance.

Be Active—Exercise is critical to increase your metabolic rate. Simply walking 45 minutes four or five times a week is very beneficial.

Monitor Progress—Keeping an exercise and food log is very helpful. It can give you a true picture of how many calories you consume daily.

Plan What You're Going to Eat—This helps you to avoid bingeing.

Recognize the Stages of Weight Loss—When you reach the frustration stage you must realize that in order to be healthy, you will have to resolve to restrict food intake and keep exercising for the rest of your life.

Jump-Start Your Weight Loss Program—There are many natural substances that can be used to aid in weight loss (5 HTP, green tea extract, Citrin).

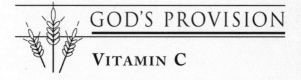

GOD'S PROVISION

VITAMIN C

Vitamin C is an essential element in producing collagen, which is the building block of cartilage. Vitamin C also inhibits the release of histamine. There are now over forty studies that indicate vitamin C can help prevent respiratory infections, nasal congestion, bronchial spasms, and other allergy symptoms due to its effects on histamine.

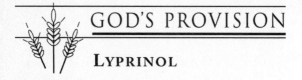

GOD'S PROVISION

LYPRINOL

Lyprinol, made from a sea mussel, recently began appearing in health food stores. Lyprinol, which is a form of omega-3 fatty acid, blocks an inflammatory enzyme known as LOX. This is very similar to the COX enzyme inhibitors, a new class of arthritic drugs.

THE SUMO WRESTLER'S GUIDE TO WEIGHT LOSS

Sumo wrestlers have discovered some proven techniques to put *on* weight. I recently did a study of these people to see what techniques they use, so that those who want to lose weight can avoid these things and do just the opposite.

1. Never Eat Breakfast—Studies show people who consume the same number of calories early in the day lose more weight than if calories are eaten late in the day.

2. Eat One Big Meal in the Evening— The body thinks it is starving and will slow down your metabolism. Eat several smaller meals earlier in the day to lose weight.

3. Eat a Big Meal and Take a Nap—Stay active. A long nap after eating can really help put the weight on.

4. Eat a Big Snack Just Before Going to Bed—Again, it's the late evening calories that can contribute to a larger weight gain.

5. Exercise Only in Short Bursts—Short periods of exercise will not increase your resting metabolism rate. It takes 45 minutes to one hour of continuous exercise (such as brisk walking) to give your metabolism a boost.

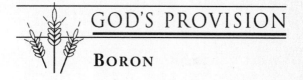

GOD'S PROVISION

BORON

Boron is a natural supplement that is showing promise in treating arthritis. This trace mineral has been shown in small clinical studies to result in significant improvement in a small number of patients with osteoarthritis.

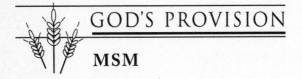

GOD'S PROVISION

MSM

MSM (methylsulfonylmethane) has been attracting a lot of attention. MSM is a stable source of sulfur and is actually a breakdown product of DMSO (dimethyl-sulf-oxide), which has been used for years by horse trainers. MSM can be helpful for osteoarthritis because it helps form certain essential amino acids such as methionine and cysteine. This sulfur is available and useful for treating the cartilage.

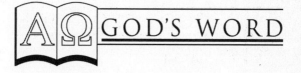

GOD'S WORD

And God said, "See I have given you every herb that yields seed which is on the face of all the earth, and every tree whose fruit yields seed; to you it shall be for food."

—Genesis 1:29 NKJV

"Every moving thing that lives shall be food for you. I have given you all things, even as the green herbs."

—Genesis 9:3 NKJV

THE MEDITERRANEAN DIET

The Mediterranean Diet is very similar to the diet outlined in Genesis 1:29 and 9:3. It seems that the diet followed by people living along the Mediterranean Sea results in some of the lowest rates of colon cancer, breast cancer, and coronary heart disease in the world. It is no accident that Israel is one of these Mediterranean countries.

THE MEDITERRANEAN DIET

Foods Consumed Daily

- *Olive Oil:* Replaces most fats, oils, butter, and margarine. It is used in salads and in cooking. It raises levels of the good cholesterol and may strengthen immune system function. Extra-virgin olive oil is best.
- *Breads:* Not sliced white bread, or even wheat, but dark, chewy, crusty breads, like rye or barley.
- *Pasta, Rice, Couscous, Bulgur, Potatoes:* Pasta is often served with fresh vegetables and herbs sautéed in olive oil. Brown rice is preferred over white. Couscous and bulgur are forms of wheat and are prepared in the same manner as rice.
- *Grains:* Eat bran cereals.

Dr. Cherry's Little Instruction Book

- *Fruits:* Eat at least 2 to 3 pieces of raw fruit every day.
- *Nuts:* Almonds or walnuts (10 per day) rank at the top of the list.
- *Vegetables:* Dark green vegetables are prominent, especially in salads. Eat at least one of the following daily: cabbage, broccoli, cauliflower, turnip greens, or mustard greens. And one of these daily: carrots, spinach, or sweet potatoes.
- *Cheese, Yogurt:* Cheese may be grated on soups or a small wedge may be combined with a piece of fruit for dessert. Use the reduced-fat varieties (2% fat or less); the fat-free often taste like rubber. Fat-free yogurt is best.

THE MEDITERRANEAN DIET

Foods Consumed Two to Three Times Weekly

- *Beans:* Pintos, great northern, navy, kidney ($1/2$ cup, three or four times weekly). Bean and lentil soups are very popular.
- *Fish:* The healthiest are cold-water fish: cod, salmon, and mackerel. Trout is also good.
- *Poultry:* White breast meat is best. Always remove the skin.
- *Eggs:* Eaten in small amounts.

THE MEDITERRANEAN DIET

Foods Consumed Two to Three Times Monthly

- **Red Meat:** Use only lean cuts with fat trimmed. Can be used in small amounts as an additive to "spice up" soup or pasta. The severe restriction of red meat in the Mediterranean diet is a radical departure from the American diet but is a major contributor to the low cancer and heart disease rates in these countries.

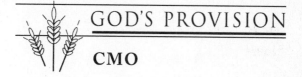

GOD'S PROVISION

CMO

CMO (cerasomal-cis-9-cetylmyristoleate) has also received some attention in research circles. This is actually a fatty acid ester discovered by Dr. Diehl at the National Institute of Health. This compound has not been studied extensively, but early studies indicate that it may help prevent the further development of arthritis. CMO is available in a capsule form.

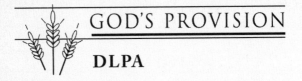

GOD'S PROVISION

DLPA

DLPA (DL-phenylalanine) has become available at health food stores and works well for the simple relief of pain. This is a form of amino acid found in foods such as peas and lentils. DLPA works by increasing endorphins, a natural pain-killing substance produced in the brain.

HOW TO SHOP FOR FOOD—WHAT TO BUY AND WHAT TO AVOID

Produce

- Most selections are a good choice in this category.
- Romaine lettuce is the best variety of lettuce.
- Peppers, tomatoes, broccoli, cabbage, potatoes, greens, cantaloupe, honeydew, kiwi, strawberries, and citrus fruits are good sources of vitamin C.
- Select deep-colored green, yellow, and orange vegetables for vitamin A, such as spaghetti squash, yellow squash, zucchini.

HOW TO SHOP FOR FOOD—WHAT TO BUY AND WHAT TO AVOID

Deli

- Sliced roast beef or turkey. Purchase the 97–98 percent fat-free variety.
- Canadian bacon is low in fat, but high in sodium.
- Avoid hot dogs; even turkey and chicken varieties are high in fat. Try a vegetarian version.

HOW TO SHOP FOR FOOD—WHAT TO BUY AND WHAT TO AVOID

Dairy

- Plain nonfat yogurt is a perfect sour cream substitute.
- Choose low-fat cheese with less than 5 grams of fat per ounce. The best varieties are Swiss, mozzarella, scamorze, ricotta, and nonfat cottage cheese.
- Use $1/2$ percent or skim milk. Buttermilk is low fat.
- Use healthy margarines (Benecol) in small amounts, preferably the nonfat variety. Extra-virgin olive oil is a good substitute.

HOW TO SHOP FOR FOOD—WHAT TO BUY AND WHAT TO AVOID

Breads and Cereals

- Whole wheat and whole grain breads, dark crusty breads (rye, oat bran, oat nut).
- It's best to combine wheat bran and oat bran cereals. Wheat helps protect the colon, while oat lowers cholesterol.
- Watch out for granola; it usually contains too much fat.

HOW TO SHOP FOR FOOD—WHAT TO BUY AND WHAT TO AVOID

Canned Foods

- Avoid fruit punches and drinks; use 100 percent pure fruit juice.
- Select canned fish with edible bones, such as salmon or sardines (but watch the salt).
- Canned beans, peas, and corn are all good sources of vitamins, minerals, and fiber. However, canned vegetables are not as nutritious as fresh or frozen. Use them only when convenience is a priority.

HOW TO SHOP FOR FOOD—WHAT TO BUY AND WHAT TO AVOID

Packaged Products

- Avoid palm, palm kernel, and coconut oils.
- Unsalted pretzels are a good low-fat snack.
- Microwave popcorn is often high in fat and salt. Air popped is the healthiest. Another healthy method of popping corn is to pop it in a heavy pot using canola oil.
- Eat potato chips only occasionally, and buy no-salt, fat-free varieties.
- Several types of dried beans lower cholesterol, including great northern, pinto, kidney, and navy.
- Long-grain brown rice is a good choice.
- Buy only cookies containing no palm or

coconut oil that have less than 3 grams of fat per cookie and no hydrogenated oils.

- Try cookies made with fruit juices and no hydrogenated oils (from the health food section).

HOW TO SHOP FOR FOOD—WHAT TO BUY AND WHAT TO AVOID

Fats, Oils, Dressings

- Extra-virgin olive oil is the best choice for salads and cooking; canola is a good second choice.
- Use low-fat, no-cholesterol cooking sprays. (You can also purchase oil sprayers that you can fill with olive oil.)
- Butter Buds can be used on potatoes and other vegetables.
- Use fat-free mayonnaise.
- Use low-fat or nonfat dressings with less than 10 calories per tablespoon. Italian dressing is great for salads and for marinating meat, poultry, and vegetables.
- Use seasoned vinegars, lemon juice, and herb/spice blends on fish and vegetables.

HOW TO SHOP FOR FOOD—WHAT TO BUY AND WHAT TO AVOID

Meat Counter

- Avoid animal fat (as much as possible) and organ meats (like liver).
- Use lean trimmed cuts: flank steak, round steak, sirloin, tenderloin, ground sirloin, ground round, ground chuck.
- Pork is generally very high in fat; tenderloin of pork is lowest (26 percent). Bacon is 80 percent fat!
- Choose "select" instead of "choice" or "prime."
- Limit or avoid ribs, corned beef, sausage, and bacon.

HOW TO SHOP FOR FOOD—WHAT TO BUY AND WHAT TO AVOID

Fish/Poultry

- Choose deep-sea fish such as salmon, tuna, mackerel, sea trout, and herring.
- Limit shrimp, lobster, and crab.
- Fresh ground turkey is a good substitute for ground beef.
- Turkey breast steaks and whole turkey are excellent choices.
- Chicken breasts are great, but half of the fat is in the skin, so "boneless, skinless" are best.

HOW TO SHOP FOR FOOD—WHAT TO BUY AND WHAT TO AVOID

Frozen Food

- Choose frozen dinners with less than 15 grams of fat, 400 calories, and 800 mg. of sodium.
- Choose frozen juice concentrates with no added sugar.
- Ice milk and nonfat frozen yogurt are better choices than ice cream.
- Frozen juice bars and fruit bars without any added sugar are great dessert choices.

FOODS THAT AFFECT THE MIND

- Seafood: Seafood is high in selenium, and studies have determined that people who do not get enough selenium tend to suffer more depression, fatigue, and even anxiety. When enough selenium is available, mood changes improve significantly. Certain nuts are high in selenium. Sunflower seeds and oat bran are good sources.

- Folic Acid: A deficiency of folic acid can lead to depression, dementia, and even psychiatric problems. Folate (folic acid) deficiency is common in the U.S. and studies show that correcting folic acid deficiency with as little as 400 mcg. daily can increase brain chemical transmitters and can correct forgetfulness, depression, and irritability. Good sources are spinach, lima beans, and leafy green vegetables (or a supplement).

- Garlic: Studies indicate that garlic tends to be a mood elevator, and people who take it regularly report less irritability, fatigue, and anxiety. Concentrated capsules equivalent to one clove daily work well.
- Peppers: A primary chemical in chili peppers (capsaicin) can cause the release of brain chemicals (endorphins) that produce a positive effect on mood.
- Caffeine: Caffeine is a widely used mood elevator taken by millions of people. Studies show it can function as a mild antidepressant through a complex effect on certain brain chemicals. Additional studies indicate caffeine can increase concentration, enhance thought processes, and reaction times. Don't exceed two cups of coffee daily. Certain people should avoid it entirely.

FOODS THAT AFFECT YOUR MEMORY

- Zinc: Slight deficiency in zinc can lead to poor memory function and mental activity in general. Regular intake of cereals, turkey, and legumes can prevent deficiencies. The amount of zinc in most multivitamins is generally sufficient to supply our needs.

- Carotene: Adequate amounts are critical to ensure proper thought processes. Good sources are dark green leafy vegetables, carrots, and sweet potatoes. Or, two 15 mg. capsules daily can supply more than enough.

- Iron: Essential to maintain normal mental function; found in greens and lean red meat. Take caution, however— excessive amounts can be toxic.

- Riboflavin: Found in almonds, cereals, and skim milk. It is helpful in maintaining memory function.

- Thiamine: Another essential substance for normal memory function. Can be found in wheat bran cereal, nuts, and wheat germ.
- Avoid animal fat: It not only increases the risk of heart disease and numerous cancers, but also alters chemical transmitters in the brain that in turn can cause memory changes and affect thought processes.

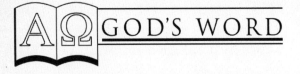

GOD'S WORD

The Lord will keep you safe from secret traps and deadly diseases. He will spread his wings over you and keep you secure. His faithfulness is like a shield or a city wall. You won't need to worry about dangers at night or arrows during the day. And you won't fear diseases that strike in the dark or sudden disaster at noon.

—Psalm 91:3–6 CEV

Dr. Cherry's Little Instruction Book

RECOMMENDED DAILY SUPPLEMENTS

Vitamin C (should NOT be time-released)	2,000 mg.
Vitamin E (should be "natural")	800 I.U.
Beta Carotene	15 mg.
Selenium	200 mcg.
Chromium Picolinate	300 mcg.
Coenzyme Q-10	25 mg.
B-100 Complex	1 tablet
Calcium (citrate, lactate, carbonate)	1,000 mg.

These represent the minimal supplements. A well-balanced, high potency multi-vitamin/mineral supplement is the most efficient, cost effective way to get your daily essential nutrients.

FIVE SPIRITUAL PRINCIPLES OF HEALING

In my medical practice, there were certain specific spiritual principles that emerged that helped lead patients toward their healing in ways we had never seen before. Through the leading of the Holy Spirit, God directed us to review these principles with all of our patients who were seeking healing from specific problems. The following pages summarize these principles.

FIVE SPIRITUAL PRINCIPLES OF HEALING

1. *Basic Principles of Healing*

   Jesus bore our sicknesses and diseases. (See Matthew 8:17, 1 Peter 2:24, and Isaiah 53:4–5).

   Jesus is our healer.

   Satan is the source of sickness and disease.

   We can hinder our healing by improper eating, excessive stress, lack of sleep, etc.

FIVE SPIRITUAL PRINCIPLES OF HEALING

2. *Peace*

Having peace in your spirit is essential to healing.

Before you pray for healing you must deal with anxiety and fear over your illness.

Cast all your fears and worries on God (1 Peter 5:7 AMP).

FIVE SPIRITUAL PRINCIPLES OF HEALING

3. *Pathway to Your Healing*

Begin praying a different way about your healing. Ask God to reveal His specific pathway for your healing (John 9:7).

You must bind generational curses (Deuteronomy 5:9). This covers the genetic tendency of disease to be passed down in families.

FIVE SPIRITUAL PRINCIPLES OF HEALING

4. *The Power of Healing*

The power of our healing is orchestrated through the words of our mouth.

Utilize the power that's in the prayer of agreement (Matthew 18:19).

Understand the power of healing that resides within us through God's presence in the form of the "other comforter," the Holy Spirit.

FIVE SPIRITUAL PRINCIPLES OF HEALING

5. *The Persistence of Healing*

Healing is often a process. It can be instantaneous and supernatural, but it can be a process that requires persistence.

Read Mark 5:22–24, 35–42 about the persistence of Jairus, and Daniel 10:12–14 demonstrating how it took twenty-one days before the manifestation of Daniel's prayer was evident.

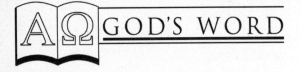

GOD'S WORD

Bless the Lord, O my soul; And all that is within me, bless His holy name! Bless the Lord, O my soul, And forget not all His benefits: Who forgives all your iniquities, Who heals all your diseases, Who redeems your life from destruction, Who crowns you with lovingkindness and tender mercies, Who satisfies your mouth with good things, So that your youth is renewed like the eagle's.

—Psalm 103:1–5 NKJV

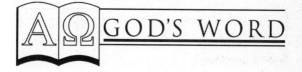

GOD'S WORD

They cried to the Lord in their trouble, and he saved them from their distress. He sent forth his word and healed them; he rescued them from the grave. Let them give thanks to the Lord for his unfailing love and his wonderful deeds for men.

—Psalm 107:19–21 NIV

How to Sleep Better

Follow a set schedule—Go to bed at the same time each night; varying your sleep pattern daily can result in a problem much like jet lag.

Exercise—Athletes have more of the deep sleep than nonexercisers. Aerobic exercise is best, but don't exercise within three to four hours of retiring.

Avoid stimulants—Caffeine (consumed after midday) will cause sleeping problems at night. Be careful with not just coffee, but also with tea, chocolate, soft drinks, and certain pain relievers.

Watch what you eat—Heavy meals eaten late can stimulate the digestive tract, which can keep you awake. A glass of milk ($1/2$ percent or skim) at bedtime really can help you sleep.

Exposure to sunlight—Sunlight exposure stimulates a chemical release that controls our awake/sleep cycle. If you can't fall asleep easily at night, experts recommend one hour of sunlight exposure in the morning.

Don't go to bed with stress—Read and do what 1 Peter 5:7 tells us: Cast all your cares on God. This is God's secret for dealing with the stresses, worries, cares, and anxieties of this world.

Cancer Is Defeated

Cancer is so limited . . .

    It cannot cripple love,
    It cannot shatter hope,
    It cannot corrode faith,
    It cannot eat away peace,
    It cannot destroy confidence,
    It cannot kill friendship,
    It cannot shut out memories,
    It cannot silence courage,
    It cannot invade the soul,
    It cannot reduce eternal life,
    It cannot quench the spirit,
    It cannot lessen the power of the
        resurrection.

                      —Author Unknown

Scripture Credits

Unless otherwise indicated all Scriptures are taken from the *King James Version* of the Bible.

Scripture quotations marked NKJV are taken from *The Holy Bible, New King James Version*. Copyright © 1982, 1994. Used by permission of Thomas Nelson, Inc., Nashville, Tennessee. All rights reserved.

Scripture quotations marked NIV are taken from the *Holy Bible, New International Version® NIV®*. Copyright © 1973, 1978, 1984 by International Bible Society. Used by permission of Zondervan Publishing House. All rights reserved.

Scripture quotations marked NLT are taken from the *Holy Bible, New Living Translation*. Copyright ©1996. Used by permission of Tyndale House Publishers, Inc., Wheaton, Illinois 60189. All rights reserved.

Scripture quotations marked CEV are taken from *The Contemporary English Version*. Copyright ©1995 by the American Bible Society. All rights reserved.

Scripture quotations identified AMP are from the Amplified Bible. Old Testament. Copyright © 1965, 1987 by the Zondervan Corporation. The Amplified New Testament. Copyright © 1958, 1987 by the Lockman Foundation. Used by permission.

BOOKS BY
REGINALD B. CHERRY, M.D.

GOD'S PATHWAY TO HEALING:

Digestion

Herbs That Heal

Joints and Arthritis

Menopause

Prostate

Vision

Dr. Cherry's Little Instruction Book

To contact Dr. Cherry or order his books

Reginald B. Cherry Ministries, Inc.
P.O. Box 27711
Houston, TX 77227-7711

1.888.DRCHERRY

www.drcherry.org

To order Dr. Cherry's all natural supplements
Mention service code K264

Natural Alternatives
Customer Service Center
P.O. Box 109
Akron, OH 44309-0109

1.800.339.5952 (orders only)

www.AbundantNutrition.com